Tea Cleanse
Rid Toxins, Lose Weight & Boost your Metabolism by Introducing Tea into your Lifestyle

Table of Contents

Introduction

Chapter 1: Toxins

Chapter 2: Detox 101

Chapter 3: Tea Cleansing

Chapter 4: Other Great Detox Teas

Chapter 5: Teas And Weight Loss

Conclusion

Introduction

We live in a world that's very toxic to our physical health. As a result, serious medical conditions such as cancer, among others, continue to become more and more prevalent compared to generations ago. As such, it's easy to feel anxious about our health. "Will I be next?" is the question often asked these days in response to news of a friend or loved one being afflicted with a serious medical condition.

We need not feel that way. Instead, we can feel hopeful that we won't follow suit. How? Through detoxification or detox. In particular, detoxing by drinking tea. In this book, you'll get a clearer picture of what detox really is by first understanding what toxins are. After learning what detox is, you'll learn a relatively simple tea cleanse routine for detoxing. You'll also learn some of the best teas for detoxing and as a bonus, you'll learn the best teas for losing weight. Weight loss is another great way to reduce major health risks and teas are excellent weight loss agents.

So if you're ready to enjoy great health via detox and weight loss with teas, turn the page and let's begin.

Chapter 1: Toxins

There's nothing new about detoxification – detox for short – diets. In the last several years however, there has been a significant rise in the public's interest on the topic to the point it's become en vogue again. Everything from powders, pills and juice cleanses has grown the real definition of the word into something that's already far from the original intended one. Even exercising has already jumped on the detox bandwagon with tag-lines such as "sweat the toxins out" or "sweat detox". And adding to the growing confusion on detoxification are testimonies on the efficacy or potency of the latest detox diets by celebrities and paid ads.

Caution must be taken here as we tread on the ground called detoxification. In particular because many of today's "detox" programs don't really understand what toxins are and how such toxins can cause much harm to our bodies, among other things. Unless we clearly understand what toxins are, it's practically impossible to evaluate whether or not a particular detox program is effective or not. That's why before embarking on a detox program and potentially wasting good money, we need to first understand the core of what detoxification programs are all about – toxins. Only then can we truly understand what detoxification really means.

TOXINS

To cut through all the ambiguity that surrounds the word, many of which are intentional, let's go to how the dictionary (thefreedictionary.com) defines it:

1. A poisonous substance, especially a protein, that is produced by living cells or organisms and is capable of causing disease when introduced into the body tissues but is often also capable of inducing neutralizing antibodies or antitoxins.

2. A poisonous or harmful non-biological substance, such as a pollutant.

In layman's terms, toxins are harmful stuff. The reason why these definitions sound a bit vague, ambiguous or general is because toxins come in different kinds, each with varying harmful effects on the human body. But to be clear on the topic for purposes of our discussion, let's classify them into internal, external and behavioral.

Internal Toxins

Our bodies are indeed wonders of creation. It can defend, repair and also poison itself. Our bodies, as a natural consequence of functioning normally, produce internal toxins. But don't worry – our bodies also have built in mechanisms that help flush out such (natural) toxins and keep them from building up critical mass.

How do our bodies produce natural, internal toxins? The process of burning energy to repair or replace damaged or dying cell tissues – also referred to as metabolism or the metabolic process – results in the creation of waste materials or internal toxins that our bodies need to break down, recycle and dispose of.

Generally speaking, internal toxins are in and by themselves not really that dangerous. What makes them so, however, is accumulation. As our bodies continuously produce toxins, they don't get the chance to take care of the toxins that accumulate over time. What happens instead is that such toxins are merely put aside – like what we do to emails of less urgency – and continue to accumulate to a point where they can be damaging to the cells and organs that surround it. Without the necessary assistance, these toxins can obstruct our natural body systems and make our bodies work harder and burn more energy to continue functioning normally. Burning more energy can create more toxins and the cycle just perpetuates itself.

Some of the things that can significantly affect our bodies' levels of internal toxins include basic medicines like proton pump inhibitors, which are standard for people suffering from acid reflux. This type of medicine, as with other antacids, can affect the digestive system to the point that it slows down and prevents our bodies from fully absorbing vitamins and minerals. Other ordinary everyday medicines like Tylenol are believed to interfere with our liver's normal detoxification process and consequently, is thought of as one of the biggest reasons for liver failure.

So how can we tell if our internal toxins have already accumulated too much? The following are symptoms of such:

1. Persistent infections like chronic dysbiosis of the intestines or sinusitis;

2. Delayed and immediate allergic reactions, most common of which include corn, eggs, dairy and gluten sensitivities; and

3. High levels of liver enzymes.

External Toxins

If we think of our bodies as if they were very efficient machines, why then do we become toxic? The answer is very simple: it's not just our bodies that create the toxins it suffers from. In short, toxins can also be produced outside our bodies and these can be absorbed or ingested.

It's easy to get caught in the trap of believing that external toxins only come from the stuff we eat, especially when we listen to many celebrity health "gurus". Because of the great focus and interest in genetically modified organisms (GMOs) and other similarly unhealthy food ingredients, it's so easy not to notice the ordinary everyday products that contain toxins. The truth is, external toxins can also be acquired through the use of ordinary everyday products such as cosmetics and even drinking water. Some of the most common external toxins and their sources include:

1. Aluminum content of antacids, deodorants and antiperspirants;

2. Bad air inhaled inside poorly ventilated enclosures or those with inefficient air filters, which can lead to what's called "Sick Building" syndrome;

3. Debris, smog and smoke;

4. Harmful chemicals present in many pet products and household cleaners;

5. Lead from canned goods, blinds and old paints;

6. Mercury in fish like tuna;

7. Molds, which can be breathed in when in basements, bathrooms or other poorly ventilated enclosures;

8. Phthalates and Bisphenol A in many soft plastic products; and

9. Ultraviolet radiation from the sun.

Behavioral Toxins

Remember how toxins come in various forms or kinds? Toxins aren't just limited to "physical" ones such as the external or internal – it can also be behavioral. In particular, we're talking about attitudes, actions and behaviors that can result in increased production of internal toxins. Case in point: always working long and hard hours at the office. Such a chronic behavior and others like it can add up to the point where it can become toxic for our health.

Chronic stress is just as toxic as taking pain Tylenol on a daily basis. Stress per se isn't bad for the health. What we're talking about here is chronically excessive stress that can lead to undesirable changes in the way and what we eat, our energy levels (lethargy), as well as mental issues like depression and anxiety disorders.

Other examples of behavioral toxins include:

1. Excessive and unhealthy eating;
2. Poor self-control;
3. Sedentary lifestyle;
4. Smoking; and

Substance addiction (alcohol, drugs, etc.).

Chapter 2: Detox 101

Now that we have a clear picture of what toxins are, we are in the position to understand what a detox really is. Referring to thefreedictionary.com, again, detox is defined as "treatment designed to rid the body of poisonous substances...". And if you remember from the previous chapter, our bodies have the natural mechanisms to detox itself, i.e., rid itself of poisonous or harmful substances. Why then, the need for a detox diet or treatment?

Let's begin with how our bodies naturally detoxify. We have 2 primary organs that act as major detoxifiers: our kidneys and liver. Basically, think of them as the primary filters that remove toxins from nutrients our bodies need. Let's talk about the liver first.

The liver is our bodies' first line of toxic defense and it acts the part via a 2-step process. The first step involves producing enzymes that convert toxins that are fat-soluble into intermediate ones, which are actually more dangerous to the body due to their relatively unstable form. But while this is so, it's where the second step kicks in. The liver produces enzymes that convert these intermediate toxins into water-soluble ones so it can be ultimately excreted out of the body.

This 2-step process or phases increases the risk of imbalances or build up. What do I mean by this? Think of the liver as a candy factory with the first and second phases being the candy manufacturing and packaging processes, respectively. If the manufacturing phase is much faster than the packaging one, there will be a buildup of candy – a bottleneck so to speak – at the second phase.

Intermediate toxins can build up in the same way the manufactured candies do in the candy factory example. If phase 2 isn't as efficient as phase 1, then there's a high risk of accumulation of intermediate toxins in our bodies. These built up toxins can potentially damage surrounding organs and tissues in the long run.

Once the liver has transformed the intermediate toxins into water-soluble ones, it passes these toxins on to our bodies' kidneys and gastrointestinal tracts for eventual excretion from the body in the form of urine or bowel. If the kidney is shot or is not functioning, the water-soluble toxins can build up in the body and poison the blood. If the gastro-intestinal tract isn't working well, solid waste can build up in the colon and if it persists over the long term, it can lead to colon cancer, among other dangerous medical conditions.

BACK UPS

While our bodies can be naturally efficient when it comes to detoxification, we live in a world where it can be easy to overwhelm the liver and kidneys to the point they aren't able to effectively or optimally deal with toxins. In particular, the primary reinforcements include our skin, bladder, lungs and large intestines. But because these organs aren't naturally or primarily detox agents, they need to get extra energy in order to provide the necessary back up to the liver and kidneys. But if overworked, they too can be overwhelmed and stressed to the point that their effectiveness is compromised. When this happens, toxins can still build up and over time, such buildup can cause tissue and cellular damage. Among the possible medical conditions that can arise from such are arthritis, asthma, tumors, cysts and skin irritations.

DETOX DIETS

Detox programs or diets can help our liver and kidneys do their jobs well to avoid imbalances or toxin buildup in our bodies. Contrary to popular opinion that we can simply "sweat away our toxins", the best way to detox our bodies is beginning on the inside going out. Certain types of foods are known to more effectively break toxins down while containing key enzymes that carry toxins out through our digestive tracts. Doing so helps reduce our livers and kidneys' detox burdens. As you may have already figured out by now, we'll talk about detoxification by drinking tea.

Chapter 3: Tea Cleansing

One possible reason why many people are turned off with the idea of going on a detox despite it's clear health benefits is the wrong impression that it will take up too much of their precious time and disrupt their everyday schedules. But truth is, it isn't hard at all. It's even possible that many such people, some of us included, are already into the detox process simply by downing this stuff regularly – and I'm talking about tea! And in particular, green tea.

How is this so? Consider the reason why many health enthusiasts, professional or otherwise, refer to green tea as some sort of health potion: it's chocked full of vitamins and anti-oxidants, the latter being known to be a key ingredient in the war against sicknesses like cancer. Green tea's key health benefits include, among others:

1. Fat Burning: Green tea's antioxidant payload helps increase our bodies' metabolism, which leads to more calories burned even while in a state of rest.

2. Stronger Immunity: The same anti-oxidant payload gives our immune systems a much-needed boost in today's polluted and toxic world.

3. Medicinal Benefits: Again, its rich anti-oxidant content has been reported to help lower risks for

specific, degenerative and neurological medical conditions such as diabetes, arthritis, Alzheimer's and specific types of cancers.

While these health benefits are already enough for many people to consider green tea a wonder or super food (or drink), forgive me for sounding like those cable TV infomercials when I say "but wait...there's more!" There's a particular type of tea that possess possibly 10 times more health bang for the buck than green tea – Japanese Matcha powdered green tea! It is believed that literally, drinking a cup of this stuff is equivalent to drinking 10 cups of regular green tea! Is that powerful or is that powerful? I thought so!

If you're not familiar with Matcha tea, it's one that's immensely popular in Japan and is starting to become so all over the world, particularly because it's a staple in many detox programs. Matcha tea's health benefits include, among others:

1. Cancer Prevention: It's chock-full off catechins, a particular kind of anti-oxidant that looks for and attacks free radicals inside the body.

2. Lower Cardiovascular Risk: It helps reduce bad cholesterol (LDL) levels.

3. Fat Burning: It can increase thermogenesis – the process of using body heat to burn fat – by as much as 43%.

4. Improved Neurological Function: Compared to regular green tea, Matcha green tea has 5 times more L-theanine, which is an amino acid that's crucial of optimal neurological functioning.

THE TEA CLEANSE

Green tea detox is made up of 2 parts: the morning refresh and the evening cleanse. Let's talk about the morning refresh first.

The Morning Refresh

This is all about replenishing lost electrolytes and vitamins from the previous night's evening cleanse. Without this morning refresh, we won't be able to enjoy the full benefits of this green tea cleanse or detox.

The morning refresh tea should preferably be one that is loaded with vitamins and anti-oxidants. And what better tea for this than the Matcha green tea! To up the refresh benefits even more, consider including healthy ingredients like spirulina, barley grass, ginseng or acai berry. But remember, these are just additions. The star of the morning refresh show is still the green tea.

Oh, when adding these other ingredients, don't expect to enjoy great flavors. Remember, it's all about health and replenishment at this point, not pleasure. But if you really need to change the tea's flavor, you can consider adding lemon juice, ginger powder, mulberries, honey or natural stevia sweetener.

The Evening Cleanse

To enjoy a full body tea detox, it's important to cleanse our bodies of the gunk, metals and toxins that accumulate daily. And similar to the morning refresh, the evening cleanse tea – also called the colon cleanse – must feature a crucial laxative ingredient – senna leaves. One great thing about using senna leaves for colon cleanses is that the US-FDA has allowed the use of senna as a natural laxative.

As with the morning refresh, drinking tea made from senna leaves is by itself a great way to cleanse the colon and adding other great natural ingredients can make it even more so. These ingredients include:

1. Dandelion plant
2. Dried orange peel
3. Lemon grass
4. Liquorice root
5. Nettle leaf

These ingredients don't just give your evening cleanse tea flavor, they maximize the health benefits and effects of your colon cleanse.

HOW TO DO THE TEA CLEANSE

The tea cleanse is one that's both effective and easy to do. First thing in the morning after hopping out of bed, boil drinking water. Put lemon juice or slices together with ginger in the just boiled water, which will help jumpstart metabolism and wake up the organs. Within 20 minutes after drinking the lemon-ginger water, drink your morning refresh tea that we covered in an earlier section in this chapter. This morning refresh tea will help the body stock up on much-needed vitamins and anti-oxidants for the day as well as a great energy boost.

As you go through your day, drink several cups of green tea, better if the Matcha type. A good guide is to drink anywhere from 3 to 6 cups throughout the day. And as you wind up your day, brew your senna leaf tea and drink before calling it a night.

You'll start to feel the cleansing benefits when you do this cleanse for 7, 14 or 28 day intervals, i.e., do this for 7, 14, or 28 days per cleanse. For this to work optimally, you'll also need to watch what you eat. If you eat toxin-laden junk foods during the cleanse, you'll just be replenishing the toxins you flush out – even more! So wise up and eat healthy during the cleanse – and even after it!

See, it's not anywhere near complicated or hard isn't it? The tea cleanse is something that can be easily incorporated in our daily routines and as such, we have no excuse for putting it off.

Chapter 4: Other Great Detox Teas

While green tea, especially Matcha, and senna leaf teas are optimal for tea cleansing, there are other teas that are also good for helping us cleanse our bodies of toxins. In this chapter, we'll take a look at some of them.

GINGER TEA

Ginger teas are considered to be great cleansing roots. They can be good drinking treats when teas are made out of them. While the taste of ginger can be a bit strong for the average person, it is gentle on the body. As such, we can drink ginger tea frequently during the day for extended periods of time.

Ginger tea – as a detox – is something that you can enjoy in the morning, can help boost your energy after lunch, or help you enjoy warm evenings during the winter or other cold nights. Being chock-full of anti-ulcer, anti-inflammatory and anti-oxidant compounds, ginger teas are hands down one of the best teas for cleansing and overall health.

Ginger is a good detox agent due to its ability to improve circulation, stimulate digestion and help our bodies flush out toxin via sweat. It's also helpful in keeping toxin buildup in the liver and colon in check.

BURDOCK TEA

Though not as popular as green tea or other tea superstars, burdock is a very powerful detox agent. It's been used in blood purifying activities for hundreds of years, particularly through its diuretic effects that help the body flush out toxins via urination.

Burdock tea contains a compound called polyacetylene, which has antifungal, antibacterial and electrical conductivity properties. Aside from helping clean the blood, this compound is known to increase circulation to the skin, which helps detoxify the body's epidermal tissues.

The roots of the burdock herb also help strengthen the immune system while cleansing the blood. Burdock also helps improve digestion and the liver's functioning. These two processes are important in the body's natural efforts to flush out toxins everyday. A cup of burdock tea a day can help in the detox process and improve the way we feel.

RED CLOVER TEA

This tea's capacity for detox is due to its high amount of antioxidants, which is quite popular for the ability to fight cell-damaging free radicals in the body.

The good thing about red clover is that it can pretty much grow anywhere, which makes it very easy to find them for brewing a good cup of cleansing tea. In particular, the most useful part for detox and medicinal purposes is the flower. Drying up the flowers can help preserve it for up to a year or even longer. And if you're not up to looking for red clover for brewing tea, you can easily buy organic red clover tea for easy detox and strengthening of the immune system.

Traditionally, red clover has been – and continues to be – used to detoxify the liver and the blood. It's also a good expectorant, which helps cleanse the lungs of phlegm and other toxins.

CAYENNE PEPPER TEA

More and more people are including cayenne pepper in their diets as word about its health benefits continue going around. As a spice, it can be directly added to delicious dishes. But to enjoy a more direct and potent detox or cleansing effect, it's better to brew it as a tea.

How does cayenne pepper help detox the body? It does so by stimulating our bodies' circulatory system, primarily by helping open up the capillaries, improving digestion and regulating blood sugar. And while cayenne pepper can lead to a runny nose, blowing the nose helps clear mucus that carries toxins. Cayenne pepper is also a naturally antifungal and antiviral food that can help us stay healthy via a strong immune system.

The best way to enjoy cayenne pepper tea is by mixing 1/8 teaspoon of cayenne pepper in hot water and lemon juice and drinking the stuff every morning.

MILK THISTLE TEA

What makes this tea a winning one is its liver benefits –
and we know that the liver is one primary way our
bodies detoxify naturally. Boost the liver and we boost
our detox.

Milk thistle is also great for maintaining a good
performing digestive system, which is of great help to
the liver when it comes to flushing out toxins from the
body. In particular, silymarin is the active ingredient in
milk thistle that naturally supports and protects our
livers. Milk thistle extracts have been reported to be of
great help to people suffering from liver conditions.

When going for milk thistle tea, go for those that contain
at least 80% silymarin.

CILANTRO TEA

More than just one of the best culinary herb out there,
cilantro is also a good detox agent that can help flush
out toxins from the body. In particular, it helps us detox
by promoting a healthy digestive system for efficient
and regular urination and bowel movements.
Remember the candy factory assembly line analogy
from earlier?

Just how good is cilantro as a cleansing agent? Consider
the fact that it can be used to purify water! If it can do

that for water, how much more can it do for our bodies, eh?

Cilantro contains great healthy stuff like active phenolic compounds, flavonoids and phytonutrients, among others. But its most powerful compounds are linoleic acid, cineole and dodecenal. Linoleic acid and cineole are excellent for addressing rheumatoid arthritis while dodecenal is used to fight bacterial infections and for removing harmful microbes from our bodies.

But since we're talking about detox, I saved the best for last – cilantro is also popular because of its ability to remove from the body heavy metals. Drinking a cup or two of cilantro tea daily can help your body in its detox efforts and help you feel more energetic.

GARLIC TEA

This tea is possibly the riskiest of detox teas. It puts you at high risk of becoming un-kissable because it can make your breath smell like garlic. But hey, being kissable and sick is worse than being un-kissable and healthy! But the best thing is to be both kissable and healthy.

Seriously, garlic is one of nature's most potent foods (health wise). It's great for cleansing the body and providing it with key nutrients. It also offers good liver function support, which translates to better natural detoxification.

To enjoy garlic tea, which can help reduce your risks of being bitten by a vampire, simply boil 3 cloves of garlic (sliced in half) in 3 cups water. As soon as the water starts to boil, remove from heat and mix in ½ cup of honey and ½ cup of lemon juice. Strain to remove solid particles like the garlic before enjoying. Drink up to 3 half-cup servings daily.

DANDELION TEA

It helps the body detoxify by increasing enzymes that help in the detox process. It's even believed to assist in the removal of certain carcinogens. As such, dandelion tea is another good tea for detoxing and for good overall health.

Dandelion is a good way to spring-clean the body as it supports and stimulates the liver's function as well as improving the function of the gallbladder. Dandelion tea is also an excellent diuretic, which helps the body flush out toxins better via urine. It's also great for digestive tract cleansing. Dandelion tea is believed to be especially helpful in reducing the risks for gallbladder and kidney stones. And lastly, it helps in cleansing the skin from within by hindering bacterial growth.

It's best to enjoy dandelion tea on an empty stomach every morning in order to maximize cleansing of the alimentary canal, relieve constipation and address digestive problems.

CHICORY TEA

Similar to cilantro, chicory tea assists the body in flushing toxins out by stimulating the production of gastric juices and promoting a healthy digestive system. It's sometimes referred to as blue sailor, blue dandelion, endive, cornflower and succor. Chicory is an herb that's abundant across the United States, Asia and Europe.

Chicory has a long history of being used in treating dysfunctions in the liver, often being recommended for jaundice or yellowing of the skin, which is often related to liver or gallbladder issues. When it helps promote liver health, it promotes better detox.

Chicory tea is great for detox via increased volume of urine, being a diuretic. Plus, it also helps relieve constipation and promote better bowel movement, which contributes to better detoxing or cleansing of the body.

If you're a big fan of coffee, the good news is that chicory tea tastes a whole lot like coffee – at least according to many people. Drinking chicory tea helps you hit two birds with one stone – you get your "coffee" fix and detox at the same time!

FENUGREEK TEA

This herb, which is more popular in Europe than in the United States, is especially helpful for relieving bloating or indigestion, both of which are digestive tract issues. This herb can help the liver's capacity to flush toxins out of the body, which is the primary reason it's included in this chapter. Fenugreek tea is made from the herb's seeds, which are also great for slowing down the rate at which sugar enters the blood stream.

Fenugreek is a strong laxative, which allows it to flush out toxins from the body through bowel movement. As such, you'll need to think twice about whether or not to drink the stuff before important events.

REGULAR DETOX

While detox programs or diets are generally best done thrice a year at most, drinking any of these detox teas regularly can help prevent toxins build up or at least minimize such build up. When that happens, detox programs or diets can be very effective in cleansing the body and improving overall health and well being. Remember, an ounce – or in this case, a cup – of prevention is better than a liter of cure!

Chapter 5: Teas And Weight Loss

More than just cleansing, teas can help us lose weight too! In this final chapter, we'll take a look at the best teas for losing weight.

ROOIBOS TEA

Made from rooibos leaves, a red bush plant, this tea is great for the tummy and contains powerful and unique flavonoid known as aspalathin. According to studies, this particular flavonoid compound is helpful in minimizing production of stress hormones. This is especially helpful for people who are huge "stress eaters" or those who tend to eat significantly more food when under stress. By minimizing stress hormones that trigger stress responses like overeating, the aspalathin content of rooibos tea effectively helps reduce hunger pangs.

MINT TEA

Mint tea can help you stave off cravings, especially for unhealthy snacks. In particular, mint tea can help you smell yourself to weight loss!

How's that so? Certain scents do nothing but trigger our cravings for certain types of food, such as that of cinnamon flavored muffins, trans-fat laden donuts, or pizza that's topped with just about every unhealthy ingredients known to man. On the other hand, some scents have the opposite effect – they suppress appetite or cravings!

A published study found that sniffing peppermint once every other hour led to a monthly average weight loss of about 5 pounds. While mint tea doesn't have as much caffeine, which helps burn body fat, its scent can help suppress appetite or cravings enough to aid in healthy weight loss.

WHITE TEA

This particular tea is considered to be a fat-blocking tea, i.e., it helps minimize accumulation of body fat. It's also considered to have the highest anti-oxidant content due to it being the least processed of all teas as it's naturally dried in sunlight in most cases.

The results of a published study showed that drinking white tea can help both increase and reduce lipolysis (breaking down of body fat) and adipogenesis (formation or accumulation of body fat), respectively. This was attributed to white tea's high amounts of ingredients believed to be active when it comes to body fat cells. So if you're looking for the ultimate diet tea, white tea may well be it!

GREEN TEA

No list of weight loss teas will ever be complete without green tea! Considered to be a great and natural way to boost metabolism, green tea helps break down fat cells and burn them to kingdom come!

The best way to enjoy the fat-burning benefits of green tea is to drink a cup of the stuff right before exercising. Studies have shown that compared to those who exercised without drinking green tea beforehand, green tea drinkers lost as much as 2 pounds more on average.

Catechins are the magical compounds present in green tea that gives it that metabolic edge. Catechins help trigger the breaking down of stored body fat as well as helping the liver convert such fat into energy much faster.

OOLONG TEA

This tea is a light and floral one that's similarly packed with catechins, which help promote a faster metabolism. Some studies have shown subjects losing as much as 1 pound of body fat a week by drinking oolong tea. As such, it's another great tea for weight loss.

WEIGHT LOSS TEAMWORK

While teas can help much when it comes to losing weight, it's best combined with proper nutrition and exercise. Simply put, all of its weight loss benefits can be negated by eating huge amounts of food and leading a sedentary lifestyle. To unlock these teas' full weight loss potential, it's best to combine them with a healthy diet and regular exercise. The synergistic effect of the 3 will guarantee a successful and healthy weight loss.

Conclusion

Knowing about toxins and how you can harness the natural power of teas to detox yourself and lose weight is only half the battle for great health. The other half is action. In particular, application of what you learned in this book. As such, I highly encourage you to start applying what you learned here as soon as possible. Given that the tea cleanse routine you learned here is very easy and most of the teas enumerated in this book are relatively easy to buy, there's really no excuse to put it off. And the longer you put off the tea cleanse, the higher the risk of not pushing through with it at all.

Time is gold and health is wealth. Act now and start your tea cleanse today! Here's to your excellent health!

www.ingramcontent.com/pod-product-compliance
Lightning Source LLC
Chambersburg PA
CBHW060445290526
45793CB00002B/577